NYC Health Beck & Call a State of Wellbeing

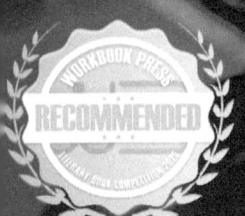

PBody Blaque

WORKBOOK PRESS LLC
187 E Warm Springs Rd,
Suite B285 Las Vegas NV 89119 USA

Website: https://workbookpress.com/
Hotline: 1-888-818-4856
Email: admin@workbookpress.com

Ordering Information:

Quantity sales. Special discounts are available on quantity purchases by corporations, associations, and others. For details, contact the publisher at the address above.

Library of Congress Control Number:

ISBN-13:   978-1-965732-22-9   Paperback Version

REV. DATE: 10/29/2024

NYC Health Beck & Call

A

State *of*

Wellbeing

By

PBody Blaque

Contents

My Disclaimer

The publisher and the author provide this book and its contents on an "as is" basis and make no representations or warranties of any kind with respect to the book or its contents. The publisher and the author disclaim all such representations and warranties including but not limited to warranties of health care for a particular purpose. In addition, the publisher and the author assume no responsibility for errors, inaccuracies, omissions, or any other inconsistencies herein.

The content of this book is for informational purposes only and is not intended to diagnose, treat, cure, or prevent any condition or disease. You understand that this book is not intended as a substitute for consultation with a licensed practitioner. Please consult your own physician or healthcare specialist regarding the suggestions and recommendations made in this book. The use of this book implies your acceptance of this disclaimer.

The publisher and the author make no guarantees concerning the level of success you may experience by following the advice and strategies contained in this book and you accept the risk that results will differ for everyone. The testimonials and examples provided in this book show exceptional results, which may not apply to the average reader, and are not intended to represent or guarantee that you will achieve the same or similar results.

Dedication

I dedicate this book to Oscar Smith-My stepdad who was like a real father, to me, as well as a mentor, & a friend.

To Josephine Smith-She did what she could with what she knew, and she was the most motherly and caring person.

Thanks. To Elizabeth Shefton - who died of dementia. A great aunt. Thanks for the memories.

To Barbara Elaine Smith, who died of Alzheimer's. Respects to a great woman.

And Dr. Claud Anderson. A great Elder in Black History!.

Introduction

Welcome, Reader!

"Squeeze-a-ma-Jintum!" That means "Miraculous!" And I'm Pbody Blaque. My name is not just a name, but a lifestyle where each letter means something: P-b-o-d-y B-l-a-q-u-e: Power by Only Doing Yourself by Living a Quality Unlimited Existence. I put together this book to help you or someone you may know on how to live a better life. Since March 2020, a lot of things about health have become obsolete. We're in this "New Normalcy," where fear, isolation, depression, obesity, and even phobias are all on the rise. I'll show you how to defeat them in my book. I'm not only the author but also a client and will show you how to be your own greatest hero. I will also mention some things in my book such as why most foods are not digested in the body; the six fatty tissues where toxins are usually found in the body; what the one thing is that's still around, plaguing us for millions of years; and what the one most important part of the body is, which must be taken care of at all cost. I'll reveal that important part of the body in a riddle: "I have billions of eyes yet I live in darkness. I have millions of ears yet only four lobes. I have no muscle, yet I rule two hemispheres. What AM I? The answer I will reveal in a moment.

But before that…. My story starts in New York City at a place called Harlem on 135 Street and Lenox Avenue. Harlem, in general, is a place I would always migrate to because it always intrigued me and was always the place that never sleeps. What made me go there frequently was because of a class I attended at a college. It was a Black History Class that was banned because a scholastic community felt it was unnecessary and many students refused to go, but a handful of us were curious and went anyway. By the way, the answer to the riddle that I gave earlier is The Brain. It has billions of optic and auditory nerves, four lobes, and two hemispheres, and it's the only thing that can either be your worst enemy or greatest ally. The black history class I attended was taught by a woman name Ms. Jefferies. I told her I wanted learn more on the subject. She wrote down an address, gave it to me, and said, "Never stop learning." The address was the 131st and Lenox Avenue called The Black Liberation Book Store. I didn't know that my life was going to change in history, health, and life. While coming home one day from studies, I was invited to see an aunt I hadn't seen in a few months. She was one of my favorite aunts, who was in the hospital for a number of days; I hadn't known why. I went to her family's home to see her. Her name was Elizabeth. I asked how she was feeling; in turn, she asked me who I was. It wasn't a long time that we didn't see each other, so I thought she was just kidding with me. She tended to do that. She'd watched me grow up and knew everything about me. But during talks with her, she kept asking who I was. Someone finally pulled me to the side and said that she really doesn't know me; she had dementia. That's when my life changed. I thought this was the worst thing that can happen. Someone you love one not knowing you anymore. To be honest, that incident started me on my quest to health and made me realize that it can happen to anybody, so I searched for answers to see that it doesn't happen to another loved one. But for many on my biological mother and father side, it was becoming too late—many of my immediate family were dying

one by one either in a nursing home or in a hospital. To help raise the bar to health, I began discovering answers such as the seven areas that must be tended to for your body to function properly. The four metals exposed to our body daily, which cause health problems, the best low-resistance thing you can do to feel better, etc.

My book is part autobiography, part self-help, part motivational, but all health. I always believed that everyone is my equal, especially anatomically. We may not be equal in opportunities, but we all bleed and breathe oxygen. I will mention the number one thing that can stop depression without medications, a method that can rid a trauma in minutes, how to naturally beautify the body's largest organ, foods that you shouldn't combine, and the only part of your body that should have acid, etc. I may not be a doctor, but I got a PhD in results, using myself as the experiment. Taking what's useful and leaving what's useless. Though doctors have their place, I was scared of them as a kid—I guess from me being exposed at an early age to Doctor Frankenstein and Mad Scientist movies. They gave me the impression that a hospital was a place you would go but never return. Working at a hospital as an adult, I was part right, depending on the person. A lot of things about a hospital can be scary, but I taught myself to psychologically not focus on the worst parts of a hospital and just concentrate on the matter at hand. As I was learning about health, I always believed in a basic principle: "Science is better than medicine and nature is better than science." Let me explain: H2O is water in America as it is in Africa. That's science. Every year, we have spring, summer, fall, and winter. That's nature. Now when it comes to manmade medicine, though there are some breakthroughs that we may never see in our lifetime, there's one specific reason I hate taking certain kinds of medicines, whether in injection or pill form—SIDE EFFECTS.

Read on to discover: The three foods hard to digest no matter how "healthy" they may appear to be, the six hormones that rule your body, how to make your body naturally release growth hormones to maintain youth, and the things you can take daily to rid your body of acid daily. Read on.

Why Should You Read My Book

Number One:
   I wrote it. There's No Ghostwriter.

Number Two:
   I Believe In Congruency.
   I'm not just the Author, but also a Client.

Number Three: Credibility.
   I don't just give opinions but state facts and data based on science.

Number Four:
   My methods are ageless, meaning, as long as you have a human body and not an actual ghost, you can go back to this book and get results time and time again.

Number Five:
   I t's reader-friendly, where it's easy for my target audience of ages 30 to 70 years to understand it.

Why I Wrote This Book?

For four reasons: dedication, inspiration, imagination, and determination.

Dedication:

First, to my late aunt, Elizabeth Shefton. (As a kid, I had four mothers in my life— Ellen Dickerson, Ina Mitchell, my biological mother Josephine Smith, and my favorite, Elizabeth. When she died of dementia, it wasn't going to be in vain because it made me take health seriously by knowing the consequences of every action.)

Second, Barbara Elaine Smith. Many people in New York and beyond knew her as B Smith, an entrepreneur who ran B Smith Restaurant from 1986 to 2015, and also did a TV cooking Show called "B Smith with Style," which aired from 1997 until 2012. She died of Alzheimer's.

Third, Dr. Claud Anderson. One of my mentors. His endless knowledge and struggle and spirit to never give up on Native Black Americans as well as Foundational Black Americans. He taught me to stay informed, apply what I know, and create a code of conduct.

Inspiration:

Diabetes and hypertension ran in my family, but it skipped me when I changed my lifestyle and created my own reality.

Imagination:

Throughout the pandemic, I would picture in my mind a world where people are debt-free, hate-free, and disease-free. I feel that can be a reality in 2022 and beyond. I never understood how we in society can create computers and yet can't cure cancer. How we can make the most advanced technological equipment yet we can't cure diabetes. How we can formulate artificial intelligence but cannot cure heart disease. I'm trying to bring those of the 7.6 billion people who are interested in bringing themselves closer to the playing field of better health.

Determination:

From March 2020 to the present, I've seen people giving up and seem to be like The Walking Dead. No feelings and living in fear, even as others lose their lives from ways unmentioned. I guarantee you will think outside the box after reading this book. I also will add that this book is not for everybody because not everybody likes everybody. But I'm confident this book will help that somebody to feel a better life.

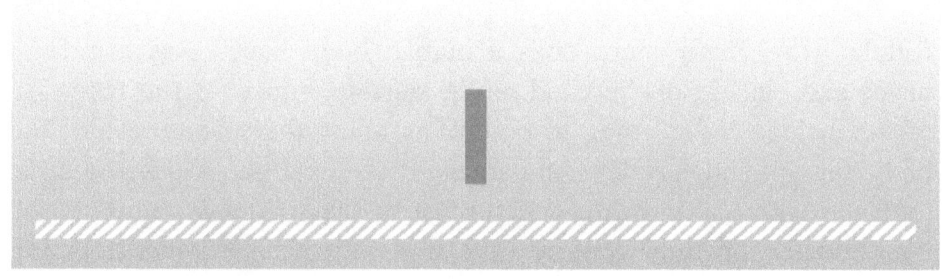

The Physical Stage

"There is a time for everything and a season for every activity under the heavens…"

Ecclesiastes 3:1

First, to be healthy long-term, you need to ask yourself what I call The Three Questions: What do you want? Why do you want it? And what are you gonna do when you get it? E.g., if someone asked you, "What do you want?" you may say, "To be healthy." Then if that someone wants you to be more specific, you may say, "I just told you, to be healthy."

"Okay. But what does healthy mean to you? Is it to be stronger? Is it to be more flexible? Is it to be disease-free? Anything is possible. Is it to have a good cardiovascular system?"

See, just psychologically telling your brain you want to be healthy doesn't tell it very much because it's vague or not specific, no more than just telling yourself you want to be rich. You must be clear with what you want and let that want be most important. You can say you want to have a balance of all these things, if you want something to come to you really fast, you've got to be a little unbalanced. You must be obsessed.

Riddle: How many sides does a human body have? Answer: Two; inside and outside. To be good on the outside, you've got to take care of the inside. We're going to be talking about the seven areas of the body (though you may say there are eight, the liver/gallbladder function together almost in unison), which must be taken care of regularly for your body to function properly. Like anything, when it comes to taking care of them, it's easy to start, but harder to continue. We are going to mention things that may be unknown to you to not only give the symptom to the problem but also help you heal the whole body. Our areas of focus are as follows:

Colon

Liver/gallbladder

Kidney

Parasite

Candida Fat Cell

Heavy Metal

Cleansing these areas alone with the suggestions provided has been known to prevent high blood pressure and diabetes.

Colon

The colon is also called the large bowel or large intestine. It is an organ that is a part of the digestive system, also called the digestive tract in the body. The digestive system is the group of organs that allow us to eat the food and use to fuel our bodies. It's the longest part of the large intestine—a tube-like organ connected to the small intestine at one end and the anus at the other. The colon removes the bad stuff—the waste/bowel—

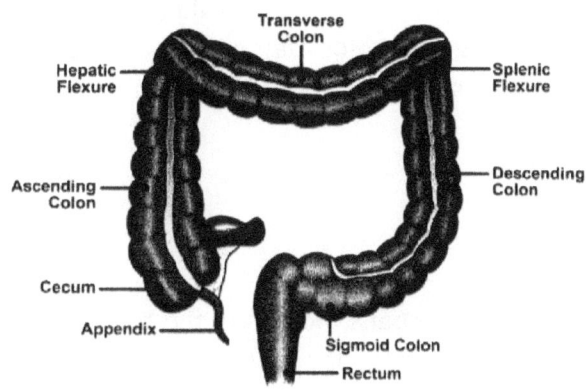

and keeps the good stuff—the nutrients. Ideally, it should be cleansed once a day. I don't recommend quick fix laxatives unless it's a last resort. If you do daily organic cleansing from well recommended companies, the body will naturally get rid of the unnecessary stuff.

The liver and Gallbladder

The relationship between the liver and the gallbladder is that your liver makes a powerful digestive juice called bile. Next, the bile passes to the gallbladder, which concentrates and stores it for later use. Bile helps

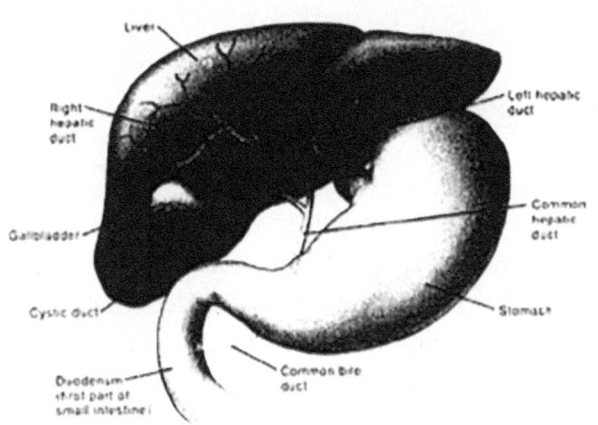

break down the food you eat. The liver is above the gallbladder and the gallbladder is a small pouch that sits just under the liver.

After meals, the gallbladder is empty and flat, like a deflated balloon. But before a meal, the gallbladder may be full of bile. The gallbladder is about the size of a small pear. Ideally, you should cleanse it every two weeks.

The Kidneys

The kidneys are a pair of organs located in the back of the abdomen or stomach. Each kidney of a person is about four or five inches long—about the size of that person's fist. The kidneys' function is to filter the blood. All the blood in our bodies passes through the kidneys several times a day. The kidneys remove wastes, control the body's fluid balance, and regulate the balance of electrolytes, which are substances that become ions in solution and acquire the capacity to conduct electricity. An ion is a charged atom or molecule. As the kidneys

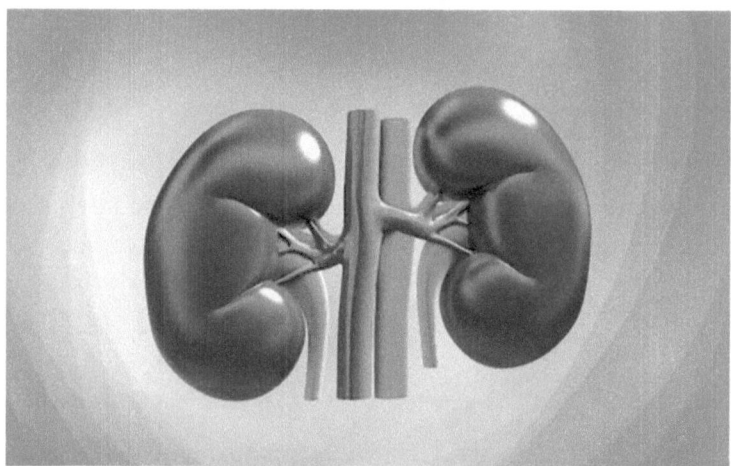

filter blood, they create urine, which collects in the kidneys' pelvis-funnel-shaped structures that drain through tubes called ureters to the bladder. The kidneys are two bean-shaped organs located just below the ribcage, one on each side of your spine. Healthy kidneys filter about a half cup of blood every minute, removing wastes and extra water to create urine. Ideally, daily cleansing can be beneficial.

Common Parasites

A parasite is an organism that lives on or in a host organism and gets its food from or at the expense of its host. It's just a living thing in another organism, which again is called the host, and often harms it while it depends on its host for survival. There are three main classes of parasites that can cause disease in humans: protozoa, Helminthes and ectoparasites. Protozoa and Helminthes largely affect the gut while ectoparasites include lice and mites that can attach to or burrow into the skin, staying there for long periods. Where do they come from? Through contaminated food such as undercooked meat or drinking unclean water. If you're eating fried foods or doing take outs often, I would recommend daily cleansing and even researching parasite zapping, which most may consider uncomfortable, but

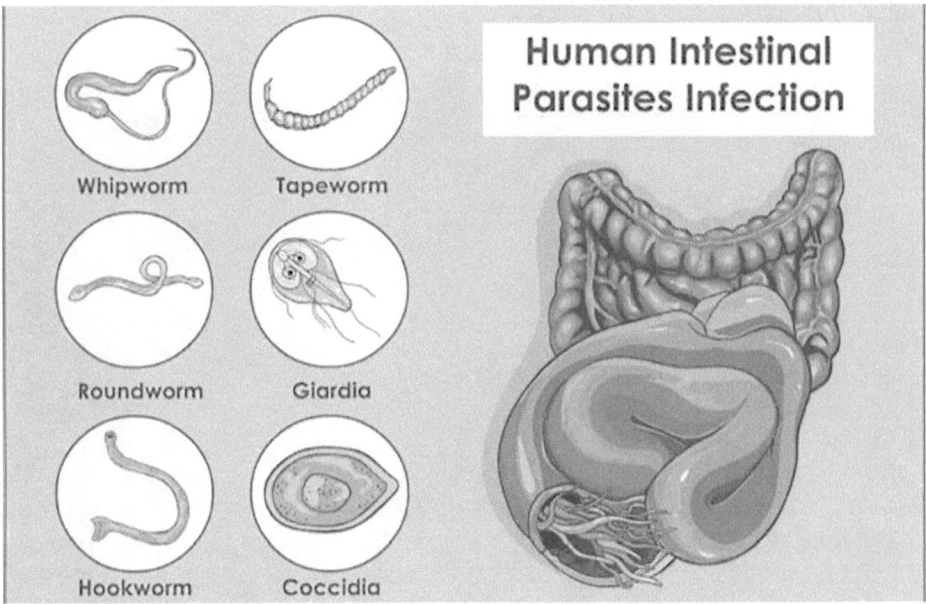

my methods are unorthodox but affective. I will further discuss this topic in another section. Ideally, you should try to cleanse them out of your system daily.

Yeast Infections

Candidiasis

Candidiasis is by far the most common type of yeast infection in human skin. Candidiasis is infection with candida species. More than twenty species of candida exist. The most common is Candida Albicans. These fungi live on all surfaces of our bodies and only occasionally cause infection. Various types of candida yeast infections are possible, including thrush, which is a candida infection of the mouth and throat. White patches appear in the mouth. Thrush occurs most commonly in the mouths of people with chronic diseases, including diabetes, HIV/AIDS, and cancer, and those who use systemic corticosteroids or other medications that can suppress the immune system. They also have been known to cause allergies. Ideally, you should try to cleanse them out daily and consistently for six weeks.

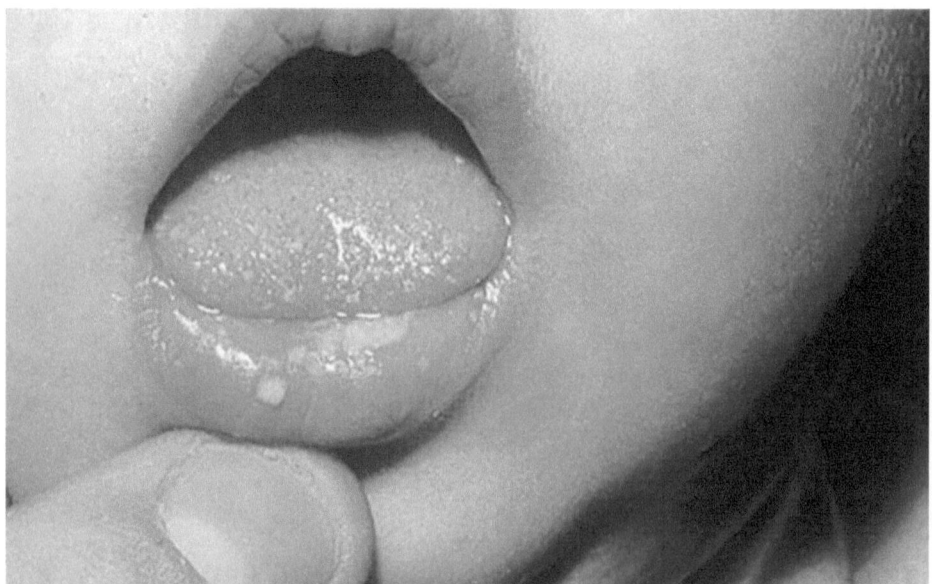

Fat Cells

There are three types of fat cells in the body: white, brown, and beige. Fat cells can be stored in three ways: essential, subcutaneous, or visceral fat. Essential fat is necessary for a healthy functional

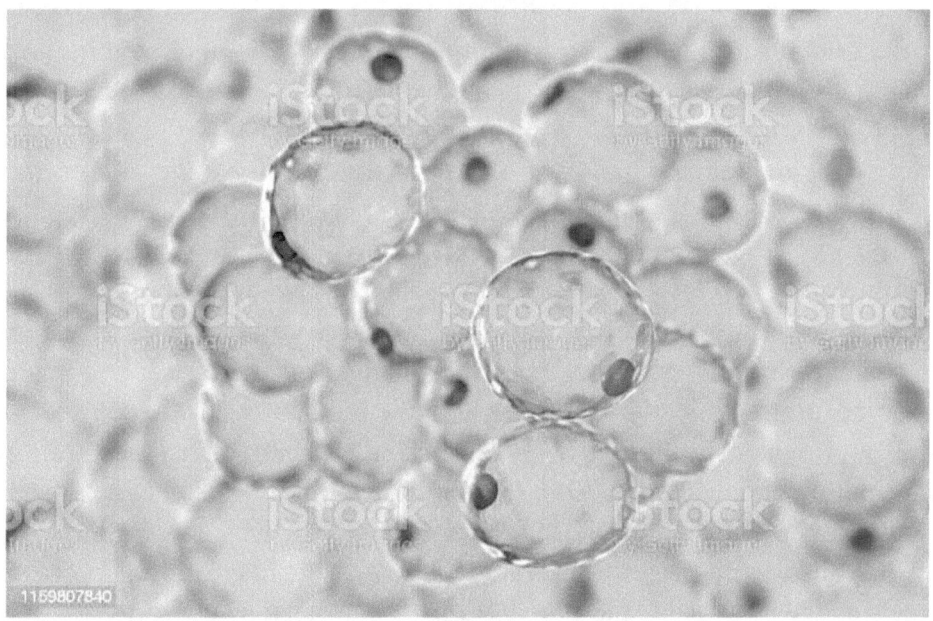

body. Subcutaneous fat makes up most of our bodily fat and is found under the skin. This is the body's method of storing energy for later use. Visceral fat is found in the abdomen among the major organs. It can be very dangerous in high levels. A high body fat percentage, and in particular, the presence of visceral fat can increase your risk for a number of diseases. Counting your calories when you eat may help you lose weight, but for the most part can drive you crazy. In my opinion, you should eat what you want but do it in moderation. Try to remember to eat a small salad before you satisfy your cravings to reduce over indulgence. There are types of fats that get a bad rap. Some may be justified because certain types of fat and the fat-like substance, cholesterol, may play a role in cardiovascular disease, diabetes, cancer, and obesity. Of course, not all fats are created equally. In my opinion, there are only two kinds: manmade and natural. But many categories of fats have two types: saturated fat and trans-fat. Saturated fats are found in animal-based foods like beef, pork, poultry, full fat dairy products, and eggs. Trans fats are in two categories: naturally occurring and artificial trans fats. Not to confuse you, but trans-fat is also called trans unsaturated fatty acids or trans fatty acids. This is found in milk and meat. I would use saturated fat in moderation. I would take the trans-fat approach with caution. Mono-unsaturated fat is a fat or fatty acid having only one double bond in their molecular structure, like olive oil, sesame oil, nuts, and red meat that are organically raised. Poly unsaturated is a fat or fatty acid having more than one double bond in their structure like sunflower seeds raw, raw pumpkin seeds, raw walnuts, and raw pine nuts. Cooked nuts have no nutritional value. I don't believe in things like vegetable oil, with the exception of olive oil because it can make oil and are technically fruits because the substance inside are seeds. LDL—low density lipoprotein—is referred to as the bad cholesterol. A normal level is less than 70 mg/dl. High levels can cause heart disease and stroke. HDL—high density lipoprotein— is the good cholesterol, which absorbs cholesterol and carries it back to the liver, which the organ then flushes out from the body. High levels of HDL cholesterol have been known to lower risk of heart disease and stroke. A normal HDL cholesterol level would be 60 mg/dl or above. Fat cells are also called adipocyte or adipose cell, which is a connective tissue cell specialized to synthesize and contain large globules of fat. Ideally, you should cleanse away excess fat cells twenty-one days every month.

Metal Toxins in the Body

Several acute and chronic toxic effects of heavy metals affect different body organs causing gastrointestinal and kidney dysfunction, nervous system disorders, skin lesions, vascular damage, immune system dysfunction, birth defects, and cancer.

Symptoms of these could be diarrhea, nausea, abdominal pain, vomiting, shortness of breath, chills, and weakness. A substance that binds to heavy metals is known as a chelator. The process that transports them out of the body is called chelation. People may also refer to a heavy metal detox as

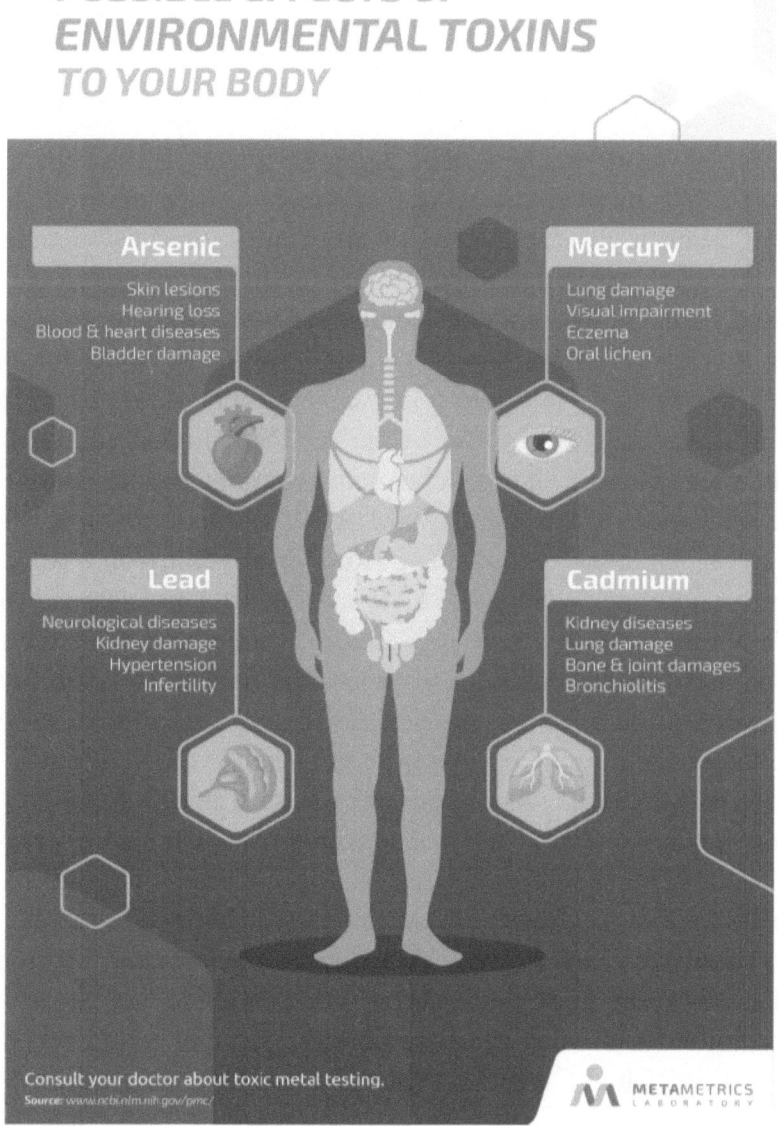

POSSIBLE EFFECTS OF
ENVIRONMENTAL TOXINS
TO YOUR BODY

Arsenic
Skin lesions
Hearing loss
Blood & heart diseases
Bladder damage

Mercury
Lung damage
Visual impairment
Eczema
Oral lichen

Lead
Neurological diseases
Kidney damage
Hypertension
Infertility

Cadmium
Kidney diseases
Lung damage
Bone & joint damages
Bronchiolitis

Consult your doctor about toxic metal testing.
Source: www.ncbi.nlm.nih.gov/pmc/

METAMETRICS
LABORATORY

Chelation Therapy. Doctors use specific chelator medications to treat heavy metal poisoning. From foods you eat, the way they're processed, to the metal fillings in your teeth, etc., causes heavy metals to be in your body. Also replacing metal tooth fillings with hard plastic would be ideal. According to various studies, heavy metal chelation using cilantro and chlorella can naturally remove an average of 87% of lead, 91% of mercury, and 74% of aluminum from the body within 45 days.

How to Make You Feel Good in Any Condition:

Eating good food that's organically grown and organically grazed is a plus. The number one cause of death is lack of food. Second cause of death is disease caused by from nutritional deficiencies in a weak immune system that's due to lack of food. Try not to eat foods genetically modified or with herbicides and pesticides. An exercise that anyone can do to relieve things like depression is by going for an hour walk during the day. Half hour going, a half hour coming back. Ideally, early in the morning at the rise of the sun. Sun's rays will go through your clothes giving a natural chemical reaction to your body. While you're walking, look at things far away. It causes a relaxing affect to the body. If you ever get a chance, experience getting on a Rebounder or Mini-trampoline. When I use to do martial arts, my classes would be held in a dance studio where they had rebounders for relaxation. This exercise helps flush toxins out of your cells lymphatic system or your cells sewage system. This is the best low resistance exercise, especially on the knees by jumping on this little thing for five, ten minutes. I also use an Inversion Table where your ankles are strapped down on a table and you slowly go upside down. The whole idea is to have you inverted where your head below your feet. You don't have to go all the way upside down, but the more you can tolerate the better. Do this for about five to twenty minutes a day to feel tremendously better. Playing your favorite songs can keep your sanity. The pandemic took away tactile contact, but hugs and handshakes can make you feel better. When I was learning Wing Chun Kung Fu, I found out about pressure points. Done

NYC HEALTH BECK & CALL A STATE OF WELLBEING

right, it can change the way you feel. The reason you may feel bad is because you're focusing on what you don't want, transmitting negative energy that opposes your happiness and blocks energy in the body; it makes you feel horrible. Try to change your focus if you feel bad. If you can't do that, try tapping pressure points. I'll explain a segment that I do, but there are many ways to do it. It's known as EFT—Emotional Freedom Technique—or TFT—Thought Field Therapy. Once you get a technique down, you just lightly tap on a series of points on the body, which takes less than five minutes to do and you just evaluate yourself to see if your stress or trauma has gone down at a scale of 0 to 10 where 0 means it's totally gone and 10 means it's there and very strong. As I've said, there are various sequences and the purpose of it is to break up the blockages in the physical body. When that bad feeling goes away, you may feel neutral.

More than anything else, the pandemic taught me to be grateful for the remainder of my life by just asking What Am I Grateful For? Now I must admit I had to practice at this one because when I came home from a stressful day at work, I would answer "Nothing!" But giving time, there's always something to be grateful for. I am a person that's not saved, but just grateful.

Tapping Pressure Points:

First, you need to identify an issue or feeling you want to get rid of. In other words, what's bothering you? How do you feel? Let's say you're frustrated. Once you identify what you're feeling, rate that feeling at a scale of 0 to 10, where 0 means there is no feeling and 10 means you have tremendous feelings. Rate the intensity or how strong that feeling is. Let's say you have an 8 intensity of feeling frustrated. Now follow this sequence or order:

First, tap the side of one hand, The Karate Chop Point, the area of your hand that you would actually give someone a karate chop on, with two or more fingers of the other. Doesn't matter which hand; just lightly tap.

Let's say you tap the left side of your left hand with the two or more fingers of your right hand. You're tapping each part of the sequence seven to ten times. You're tapping on The Karate Chop point of your left hand. Tap 10 times there. The next point is the top of your head with the first four fingers of your right hand tap on top ten times. The next point is on the right side at the beginning of the top of your eyebrow point, using two fingers of your right hand. Tap that area 10 times. Next, you tap on the right side on the bone by the eye, not the temple, using two fingers of your right hand. Tap ten times. Now tap under the right eye ten times with two fingers of your right hand. Next, tap under the nose using two fingers of your right hand ten times. Next, tap under your cleft indent above your chin, below your lower lip, ten times. Now take your right hand, make a fist, and light tap on your collar bone under your neck, right on that kind of U shape of your clavicle 10 times. And finally tap the last point where you take your right hand and tap about four inches down from under your left arm pit that lines along your left breast 10 times. Pat it using the first four fingers of your right hand. Now evaluate yourself seeing if you're feeling rate has reduced, where it maybe went from an 8 rate feeling down to a 4 rating. If your feeling is down to a 0, you're done, but if you still feel frustrated but not as much, you may have to do another round or this whole sequence again to feel even more relief. Some people new to this may have to do 2 to 5 rounds to eliminate it totally. When the feeling is gone, it's typically permanent. This whole method is based on acupuncture or acupressure. For even more effect, many people do this technique together with auto-suggestion, which is an influencing of one's own attitudes, behavior, or physical condition by mental processes other than conscious thought. In other words, commanding your brain and remind your system what it is you're working on. I didn't add auto-suggestion because that's an individual preference. But I encourage you to do your own research on the subject. Your body is like a human antenna that picks up both good and bad vibrations. Each pressure point is connected to an organ where negative energy is known to be. So even if we don't know which part of the body is affected, you would do the basic points of the body by tapping a certain area to alleviate that negative feeling to leave you. You can just tap the pressure points without any auto-suggestion and still get results. What I love about it is that it works whether you believe it or not. This method is not for those faint of heart. Good luck.

I worked in a hospital in NY in an area called The Bronx from February 7, 2007 to September 23, 2021. I worked as a Patient Care Associate or PCA. I did EKG's—electrocardiograms. This is a test that allows impulses on how fast the heart is beating. I also did phlebotomy, which is a procedure in which a needle is used to take blood from a vein, usually for a laboratory testing. The staff at my hospital got more afraid losing a life each day and it got more intense during the pandemic. I remember March 2020 like yesterday. That was the same month they banned plastic bags. Many thought the world was literally coming to an end. In my mind, I would think, "It ain't over till it's over." I had my ways of coping, seeing fear as F.E.A.R.—False Evidence Appearing Real. If death would come, it would come like a thief in the night and if you lived, it would be your chance to start over. Music was my fix every day. I taught myself to be eclectic.

I would go running on my days off, just read, or just stay informed of world issues. I am a get to the point type person, so stayed away from media elaborating negativity. I would listen to all types of podcasts and news like 1010 WINS. I liked their slogan, "You Give 22 Minutes; We'll Give You the World." That was cool. I'd daydream every chance I got as well. Doing my job without taking the job too seriously. I'd reminisce when I traveled to Las Vegas, Nevada; Houston, Texas; or Philadelphia, Pennsylvania, back then. It was a much slower time. At that time, there was no mask, no hang ups, no social distancing, and no martial law. Like they say, you never miss something till it's gone. More and more of us were feeling isolated. That wasn't hard for me, me being a loner. Besides, loneliness is a state of mind. I had a few close associates with some encounters from time to time; that was good enough for me. I would have zoom meeting learning stuff. This together apart never made sense to me, but you had to play along. I remember the first time they introduced me to the N95 mask. During the demonstration of properly putting that on, people were cheering. I said nothing because I would be outnumbered. But in my mind I was thinking, "I'm not gonna be able to breath." So, I had to see how this would pander out. Zoom, Face Time, audio or text was just about the only way to communicate. Depression was many peoples number one enemy. My research showed me a considerable complexity in the association between race and mental health. The patterning of racial differences in mental health appears to vary by indicator of mental health status. For several generations, research has shown that while blacks often have higher rates of psychological distress than whites, some studies also find that whites have elevated levels of depressive and anxiety symptoms compared to blacks. And this goes as far back as 1969 to as high as high as 2008. Blacks tend to report lower levels of psychological well-being on cognitively focused measures such as life satisfaction and happiness (Hughes and Thomas 1998), but also report higher levels of flourishing than whites (Keyes 2007). Flourishing refers to the absence of psychological disorder for wellbeing.

I would wear a mask in moderation but never when I exercise. No matter what an "expert" would say, I believe the human body needs full lung capacity with no obstruction whatsoever through the mouth and to prevent carbon dioxide from developing. Cardio workouts have been known to stop depression. One of my favorite workout programs up to this day is Tae Bo Workout by Billy Blanks. I don't look for the "latest" thing, but whether it works. And his does. Obesity is climbing at an alarming rate. Staying in front of a TV or computer all day can do more harm than good. In addition to being bombarded with radio waves, which can put your system out of whack, it does not give your body enough activity to burn fat. If you're not going outside often, you're missing the essence of life. You need to meet the sun along with oxygen to look and feel better. No matter how "old" you are, a sedentary lifestyle can be deadly. I feel the body is meant to be active for life. Drink a liter of water a day every morning. I don't think drowning your system with a gallon of water a day. God help you if there's no bathroom nearby. Even though everyone's biochemistry is different, and regardless of the numbers, let's agree on this: Most of the planet is made of what? Water. Most of your body is made of what? Water. So what should most of your intake should be? Water soluble foods. Hopefully organic fruits and vegetables. Now there are more people than organic food, so having the chance to taste true chemical free food is a blessing. For those who binge or if you're the type of person that munches habitually, meaning, eat when you're happy, eat when you're sad, eat when you're angry, etc., then try eating a fruit or small salad before lunch or dinner to cut your appetite. Drinking water with soluble foods throughout the day alone can rid your body of unwanted fat and create you ideal weight. Not something fabricated from a BMI—Body Mass Index— calculation. That measures your body fat based on height and weight, which applies to adult men and women. I feel it's based on European standards, which is different from ethnic standards. When you look at the animals of the forest, they do just fine. Some can fly well, some can run fast, and some can swim well. I can guarantee that none of them know what the guidelines of The Food and Drug Administration or The American Cancer Society are. They follow a genetic code.

OCD—Obsessive Compulsive Disorder-—is another topic that's been said to be an epidemic. I knew someone close who had it—me. It's an uncontrollable behavior or thought that you repeat over and over. As a result, you can be a hoarder, where it's difficult to let go of certain things. A key to stop it is first paying attention of your actions. While functioning throughout the day, we forget to pay attention of our actions. The key is being aware. Things may be piling up at your home. You first have to admit you have this habit and decide you want to change it. It's not easy, but it is simple by asking why you hold on to this item or items. I decided anything I haven't seen in a year that doesn't really help me in my present, I'll toss out. I decided to live for the moment to create my future; so as a result, I tossed a lot of things away. Some people who may know you may think there's something more wrong with you, but just let'em know, "Change is good." With health, you may run into a lot of setbacks. I remember being diagnosed with Discoid Lupus, which is a skin condition. The full name is Discoid Lupus Erythematosus. This is a chronic autoimmune disease affecting the skin where coin shaped lesions can form on your skin. Lesions may produce. This condition may form a rash that can get worse when exposed to sunlight. The doctor told me that it's a combination of genetics and environmental triggers. Doctors have no idea where it actually may come from, but it's not contagious. So, it made me realize it may be due to an improper diet. I eliminated pork, stayed hydrated, and combined outdoor activity. As a result, the sun stayed a friend of mine, giving me Vitamin D with no lesions.

An enlargement of the heart.

This was another challenge in my life. It's also called Cardiomegaly. It isn't a disease but refers to your heart being larger than normal when seen on an X-Ray. The most common cause of this is High Blood Pressure—stress! This occurs when narrowed arteries, which are caused by fatty deposits that build up in your arteries, prevent blood from getting to your heart. Again, the number one culprit was stress. As a kid, I was high-strung and nervous with a low self-esteem. I would have anxiety to the tenth power. I eventually picked better models of people in the world, and instead of wanting other people's approval, I decided to have my own approval first. I remember performing, doing poetry, and I asked someone how to get rid of stage fright. He was from England, and he said, "Mate, you gotta realize, you're performing in front of people who screwed up more than I did, so whatever happens, take it and adjust. Cheers!" I forgot the guy's name, but that stayed with me for life.

Cutting down on the fast food by cooking more, creating a workout routine for myself as well as discovering and relieving pressure points throughout my body helped me eliminate a lot of my stress and bought my heart back to normal. During the pandemic, I learned about a steam treatment to prevent colds and flu, which are viruses. I would do it every day. I never caught COVID-19; I was always tested negative, but I got the flu once and a cold from time to time. Learning scientific approaches helped me tremendously. For this steam treatment: Get a two to three quart sauce pan. Keep this pot you for your personal use. Fill the pot about half way with water. You can add either half a slice lemon squeezed in the water or half sliced onion for aroma therapy. This helps unclog your nose and throat. Sprinkle sea salt in the water to create a saline solution. Place it on the stove on full heat. Let it come to a boil. Once it's boiling, reduce the fire to about medium. You stand over the steam as close as possible without burning yourself and just inhale and exhale through your throat and nose. Alternate. You would do this for twenty minutes. It loosens the mucus and phlegm. I do this treatment any time I feel stuffy. Something happened to me years ago where I couldn't sit for long periods. I literally would have to stand all day for relief. The doctor's diagnosed me with chondromalacia or "runners knee." The full name is chondromalacia patella, which is a common condition causing pain in the knee cap. The Patella is covered with a layer of smooth cartilage, which normally glides across the knee when the joint is bent. Mine was damaged to the cartilage under the knee cap. The cartilage under the knee cap is a natural shock absorber. Chondromalacia patellae may develop when the knee is overused or injured. The most common symptom is knee pain, which worsens when walking up and down stairs. I would use the medication that the doctor prescribed but I would feel funny with no relief, plus I felt like a drug addict. That was the point: I didn't like medications for their side effects and decided to find a healthier alternative. I decided to meet my pain head on with knee bends. I don't know what made me do knee bends, but I would do them every day. Starting with ten knee bends a day for a month, then adding ten more each month until I got up to fifty knee bends a day. I said to myself, "If I my knees got to hurt, I'll give them a reason to hurt." But the pain would subside and I would eventually become pain-free. I also do weight training on my knees as well as use glucosamine and something called chondroitin. I found that they also help with people with osteoarthritis. They are components of the cartilage, the tissue that cushions the joints. Well! By taking them both three to six months, my cartilage felt better.

When you're getting better health-wise, you should monitor yourself anytime you feel abnormal.

Know vital signs and what they are. There are four common areas routinely monitored by medical professionals and health care providers: Body temperature, pulse rate, respiration rate, rate of breathing, and blood pressure. Although that's not considered a part of a vital sign technically it is included along with your oxygen level and is often measured along with these vital signs. For body temperature, you can take it orally (by mouth), rectally (taken in the anus, rectum, or butt, which is known to be the most accurate), axillary (under the arm), by ear (done with a special thermometer), and by skin (specifically on the forehead). 98.6 F is the average normal temperature.

The pulse is a measure of the heart rate, or number of times the heart beats per minute. The normal pulse rate is between 60 to 100 beats per minute. You can check your pulse on the side of the neck, on the inside of the elbow, or at the wrist. The respiration rate is the number of breaths a person takes per minute. You're counting how many times the chest rises. Normal rates are twelve to sixteen per minute. Blood pressure is the force of the blood pushing against the artery walls during contraction and relaxation of the heart. The range is a base between one ten over ninety (110/90) and one twenty over eighty (120/80). The high number (systolic) is when the heart contracts or pumps blood through the body. The lower number (diastolic) is when the heart is at rest and is filling with blood. The pulse oximeter is used by placing a fingertip that's attached to the machine, which measures the oxygen saturation or the amount of oxygen that's in your blood. The normal read can be between 90% for those who have sleep apnea or chronic lung disease, and 95% or higher to 100%. Any results you get when checking your vital signs or if any readings of them are not normal or abnormal, remember the one thing you must do if all else fails: Don't Panic! Let your body rest or recover after any activity then check your vital signs again. If there is still no change or your signs are higher or lower than usual, then seek medical professional help as soon as possible.

We all have twenty-four hours (the great equalizer). What you do with those twenty-four hours determines your fate. When you decide to work out or be healthier, everyone will be out to steal your time. Pick a time that is consistent and devoted just for you. Work out for at least thirty to forty-five minutes daily. Mornings are ideal, but any time you can put in is good too. As you work out regularly, you will feel a transition where you may feel sore, which is expected and normal, but if there's any searing pain that's consistent, seek medical help before it gets serious.

If you're a parent, make sure your kids are okay and within your sight if need be. Being creative to add them to your workout can be a plus, but the more time alone to focus and gather your thoughts the better. Sometimes, friends and family may feel resentful because you're doing something they can't. But if they care about you, they will eventually accept it. So decide to do it, get your equipment, find a consistent place and time, and keep the same time you pick, at least three days a week. This will give your body memory to adjust at your chosen time, and just get going. As a side note: Vitamins have been around since the turn of the century. Some may help some may not, but if you're not sure which to take, ask an experienced health professional you respect and see if they're congruent. If they recommend stuff but they don't look good or natural then that's a problem.

I experimented on myself when no expert was around and take vitamins for different reasons and would switch them often with Whole food Supplements in a concentrated form to give you the right amount of minerals, that is a chemical compound, enzymes, which are proteins that accelerate chemical reactions, and nutrients, that is a nourishment essential for life. I also try not to use synthetic vitamins over potent or organic because I feel they don't have any nutritional value at all.

Things will never be the same. Many who I knew were traumatized inside out. My heart goes out to the kids who can't have a normal life anymore and are not properly educated. It was hard for a lot of parents to get online for their children to learn from home, and God help the child that fell to the waist side and had no one. People pointing fingers how this all started.

COVID-19 is an illness caused by SARS-Cov-2. The term COVID was named by WHO, the World Health Organization. The COVID-19 acronym was derived from "coronavirus disease 2019". The name was chosen to avoid stigmatizing the virus's origin in terms of population, geography, or animal associations. SARS-Cov-2 stands for Severe Acute Respiratory Syndrome coronavirus 2.

COVID-19 was discovered in 2019. It causes people to have flu-like symptoms. With a strong immune system, you can take it like a common cold till it goes away. But a person with a weak immune and not being well to begin with could be fatal. Especially if they have other ailments in addition to COVID, like cancer, which are abnormal cells destroying your tissue; diabetes, where there's too much sugar in the blood; emphysema, which are damaged enlarged lungs, and respiratory infections, RTI, which is when microorganisms invade your tissues, causing difficulties in breathing through the sinuses, throat, airways, or lungs. When the pandemic was full blown, there was no room on the units in the hospital I worked at. It was like being on a MASH—Mobile Army Surgical Hospital— unit. Coming home from work, I would see blocks empty and shopping malls looking like ghost towns. All that the media talked about was the President or COVID and what business was next to close down. The pandemic lasted longer than the O.J. Simpson trial in 1994, which had lasted for eight months. I took online courses in business since public schools were shut down. I would have to be at work by 7a.m. What no one knew was that to keep my sane and to get rid of the stress, I would be up every morning before work at 1:30 a.m. I would train till 4:30 a.m., shower, eat breakfast, and be out the door every morning exactly at 5:34 a.m. Every day, I stayed informed with the media and read books. I never had a weight problem but was undernourished. But I went from 150 lbs. to over 180 lbs. of definition, flexibility, and strength. During the trial and error of my workouts, I found four types of workouts: muscle building, toning, cross training, and weight loss. Now, you can mix and match and incorporate your own routine but either one will give you results. You just have to know if that's the result you want. Muscle building helps increase the size and strength of your muscles. You have to push them to maximum capacity. You can only increase the size and strength of your muscles two ways: Either increase the weights or increase the "reps." A repetition or rep is one complete movement of something. E.g.: one push-up is a rep. A set is a series of repetitions. You can invest in weight gain drinks and surgeries if you wish, but I don't believe in them. You may get instant gratification with those, but long-term, those short cuts, as well as performance enhancing drugs, will do more harm than good. You will develop your own natural size if you stay consistent in your workouts. With Toning, you do this by pushing them to moderate capacity by selecting an amount of weights comfortable to you and just simply increase the number of reps. E.g.: you can complete a set of ten or twenty repetitions without discomfort, rest for a full minute, and then do another set with a minute of rest. Stay hydrated with filtered water. Weight loss you can accomplish by using a low amount of weights but increasing the number of movements or repetitions in each set. Exercise a half hour then rest thirty seconds between set. If you have a heart condition, consult with your doctor or cardiologist before you attempt any strenuous exercise. Cross training is most popular because it has variety that's a complete well-balanced workout. To do that, you don't do everything in one day; instead, you spread your routine into different days. E.g.: Maybe weight train on Mondays, Wednesdays, and Fridays. Do an aerobic exercise, like swim, run, or jog on Tuesdays and Thursdays. Then pick a complete rest day, either Sat or Sun. This is a full rest period for your body to recover or regenerate. All these activities are great for your cardiovascular system (heart and lungs). If you never worked out before, start light and avoid overdoing it. Do warm-up exercises, like stretching to circulate the blood throughout your body. Here's a muscle chart describing the important parts of the body:

Stretch before and after each workout. Stretches after workout are called cool downs, which is to bring the heart back to a relaxed state. Inhale before the actual action of an exercise and exhale during the exertion of an exercise. Try not to do the bad habit of holding your breath when lifting weights. Whether I try something or not, I'd like to research its background before I decide if it's right for me.

MUSCLE CHART

A. Sternomastoid (neck)
B. Pectoralis Major (chest)
C. Biceps (front of arm)
D. Obliques (waist)
E. Brachioradials (forearm)
F. Hip Flexors (upper thigh)
G. Abductor (outer thigh)
H. Quadriceps (front of thigh)
I. Sartorius (front of thigh)
J. Tibialis Anterior (front of calf)
K. Soleus (front of calf)
L. Rectus Abdominus (stomach)
M. Adductor (inner thigh)
N. Trapezius (upper back)
O. Rhomboideus (upper back)
P. Deltoid (shoulder)
Q. Triceps (back of arm)
R. Latissimus Dorsi (mid back)
S. Spinae Erectors (lower back)
T. Gluteus Medius (hip)
U. Gluteus Maximus (buttocks)
V. Hamstring (back of leg)
W. Gastrocnemius (back of calf)

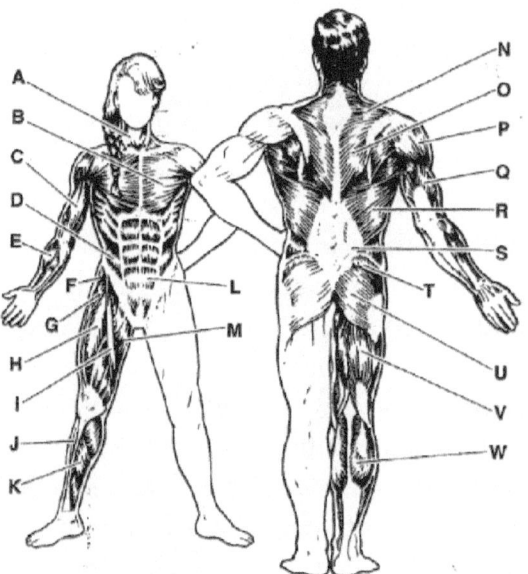

For information on the three main vaccines

Moderna: This was the first COVID-19 vaccine to come out. It was created in Cambridge Massachusetts, with the funding by the National Institute of Allergy & Infectious Diseases (NIAID). Pfizer was the second one to come out. It's manufactured by BioNTech, a pharmaceutical/

biotech company established in 1849 by German immigrants. And the third one was Janssen, which was manufactured by Johnson & Johnson and developed by Janssen Vaccines in Leiden, Netherlands, and its Belgian parent company, Janssen Pharmaceuticals.

Avoid strenuous exercise on a full stomach. Digestion is the hardest thing your body will ever do because it takes blood that you normally would need for your muscles. Once you've trained enough, your body will have memory to keep whatever level you are, but if you been away from working out awhile, like literally a month of not doing anything or you have been in an accident where you were out of circulation for some time, then you would have to start your training all over again, bringing back your passion. You may not like to work out, but seeing the good results may motivate you. You got to love yourself before you can make a move toward anything that benefits you. Start light and gradually build up. Patience is virtue. Try to find a partner to try with, maybe a soul mate or good friend who's into health as you are to train with, and spot you in case you can't lift weights or do certain routines without a partner.

Going to a gym or working out is like going to church. Though everyone may have similar beliefs, it's still a personal journey. Health can be confusing even for professionals. But realize you're going to meet different levels of aptitude and intelligence, so it's always good to know what you want first. To do that, you need to know what a lot of things in health are.

Carbohydrates are sugar molecules, along with proteins and fats that are the main nutrients found in certain foods and certain drinks. Your body breaks down carbohydrates into glucose or blood sugar, which is the main source of energy for your body's cells, tissues, and organs. It was the health trend in the twenty-first century. Seeing relatives die from medications made me decide to use a common sense approach by taking what's useful and leaving what's useless. People are living longer, but they're in so much pain that they lose the motivation to go on. Many are waiting for organ donors because their organs are failing.

Health is a billion-dollar industry, along with agriculture, tourism, computers & information technology, mining, financial services, and food industry. Even pornography is booming globally. The interests of people vary. But no matter what you're pursuing, there is a universal law: Anything you fail to use, you lose. Health is no different. I learned more from the mistakes than victories of people in all walks of life. When you stop keeping your body active, it atrophies or shrinks. You're either growing or dying. There's no in between.

Now let's focus on some other things we consume. With eggs, people ask me what's the difference between organic and conventional. They both are high in cholesterol, because of the yellow egg yolk, but with conventional eggs you're also dealing with ingredients in the egg such as pesticides, herbicides, hormones, and insecticides. The way these chemicals are created in the yolks is determined by how the chickens were raised. Any animal that's confined instead of being cage-free becomes depressed and irritable, thus releasing a stress hormone called cortisol. Also, if they're not fed decent grain, they will produce whatever they eat with all the chemicals settling in the egg. Also, there are chickens that lay brown eggs called creole or mixed.

As far as milk, I believe milk is only good for the species that makes it. Cows' milk is for baby calves. Human breast milk, from a healthy female, is the best for a human baby. I knew people who said they grew up drinking milk but have false teeth and arthritis. Another myth shot to hell. I personally recommend almond milk or, if you want that skimmed milk taste, rice milk. I would approach soy milk with caution. It has been linked with abnormalities. With bread, whole grain is the best digestible. Second would be wheat bread. As far as the things you consume with health, my disclaimer that is I am not a doctor but am merely sharing suggestions of what has worked for me.

IP-6—Inositol Hexaphosphate

I use this as an antioxidant. It's found in animals and many plants and has been known to also prevent cancer by slowing down its production as it helps make your body alkaline because cancer can't survive in an alkaline state. During the pandemic, I would follow a very simple rule: "Cold kills bacteria, but produces viruses. Heat kills viruses, but produces bacteria. Thank you, science class."

Too much protein can cause weight gain, constipation, kidney damage, heart disease, and possible cancer. But on the positive, the right amount helps your body make antibodies that fight off infections and illnesses as well as keep cells healthy to create new ones. A cup of raw nuts or two organic raw eggs in supplement drinks have been known to be enough protein for a day. Another way to lose weight without even trying is to just eat nothing but fruit from 9 a.m. to 12 noon. During this time, your body goes through the elimination cycle where it gets rid of waste. That waste is unwanted pounds. You have to do this daily on an empty stomach to speed up the process and you can eat as much as you want.

The true purpose of calcium is not to build strong bones and teeth but to neutralize the acid in your body. The stomach is the only place that should have acid to help digest. Any place else is hazardous. Calcium helps remove the access acid we get from the foods we eat, the things we drink, and the stress we make. Coral calcium is very good.

The purpose of nitrogen in the body is to make amino acids in your body, which makes protein. Amino acids are molecules combined to form proteins. The air we breathe consists of 78% nitrogen, 21% oxygen, and 1% other elements. Hence, nitrogen is a gas already present in a large quantity of air. But too much nitrogen may make you sleepy.

Fiber is a type of carbohydrate that the body cannot digest, so instead, it passes through the body undigested. But fiber helps regulate the body's use of sugars, helping to keep hunger and blood sugar in check. It helps to reduce the risk of developing various health problems. A High intake of fiber has been known to lower the risk of heart disease.

Deep breathing is a big way to get rid of stress. To fully oxygenate your body, you need to breathe in while counting to twenty; then, hold the breath to a count of twenty, followed by breathing out while counting to twenty. This is the 20–20–20 segment. In the beginning, start small, breathing in while counting to five, hold the breath while counting to five, and then breathe out while counting to five. If you can at least do half the 20–20–20 segment where you do ten deep breaths (where you breathe in counting to ten, hold the breath counting to ten, and then breathe out while counting to ten) for at least ten days, your energy will be exploding, which can eliminate a lot of coffee intake. Try it for yourself.

If you follow the same diet and belief system of somebody else, then most likely you'll get the same results of that person, especially if it runs in your family. That's called developing a family trait. You're made of thirty trillion cells waiting for you to tell them what to do. To help take care of them, always read labels of all products to see what's going in your system to give your body a better chance to live. If there's something you can't pronounce, then it shouldn't be in your body.

The purest salt for your food is sodium chloride. Sea salt is a good second. Vitamin C crystals taken regularly in drinks and certain foods can help raise your immunity against colds and viruses. Vitamin B2 100 mg is good to detoxify the toxicity in many foods if you can't home cook. Lugol Iodine Solution is very good for gas and bloating. Just six drops in a half glass of water will do the trick as well as put you in a peaceful state that's non-addictive. Aloe Vera is a succulent plant species that has been known to regenerate damaged tissue. Echinacea, a plant, and goldenseal, an herb, together can fight colds. What inspired me about health was while growing up I saw massive contradictions. As a kid, I worked at a place called Tower Records, a music store, in New York. I worked with a seventeen-year-old with salt-and-pepper hair. I dated a twenty five-year-old woman with arthritis so bad she would have to take Advil Aspirin to kill the pain while doing her hair. I used to go to the Skate Key Roller Ring in the Bronx where I met a seventy-year-old man who was the best skater I've ever seen. I even had the pleasure of meeting an eighty-five-your-old playboy. True story. He lived in Asbury Park, New Jersey. He was one of my ex-girlfriends' godfather. Woman of different generations would come to clean his house, but for the most part he was independent. He would go fishing, dive, and fix his car on his own, with a cute little white and black spotted dog as his companion. He was married once but she died. It was hard to believe he was that age. I asked him what his secret was. He said, "Stay away from negative people." Good advice.

I want to talk about the topic of water. I don't use faucet water at all and I believe you should test your water.

TDS, or total dissolved solids, refers to the total concentration of dissolved substances in the water. In other words, it's how clear the water is. The TDS level number shows how much of the total dissolved solids are present in water. TDS in drinking water originates from places like natural sources, sewage, urban, run-offs, industrial wastewater, chemicals in the water treatment process and chemical fertilizer used in the garden and plumbing. Water is a universal solvent and easily picks up impurities that can absorb and dissolve these particles quickly. Water should not have a smell or taste. A lot of experts may tell you that a good TDS level for water is between 50 and 150. I disagree. In the hospital I worked in, many patients who had jaundice were tested where they had large amounts of metals, fluoride, and parasites in their system due to drinking huge amounts of water from unclean sources. You can get a TDS hand held meter to test your water and you may have to search for a really good filtration system. The average ones would have one or two stages of filtration, which remove some of the dissolved solids in the water. But I believe you can find water filters, in both water pitcher and water bottle, with a better ion exchange system, which can remove much more impurities. There should be a zero (000) read and anything like a "006" should be replaced. Any number higher and you're taking a risk. The best water to buy would be reverse osmosis (RO) water, which is removed of chemical contaminants.

This page is devoted to the one thing that's still around that has been plaguing us for millions of years, parasites. You're made up of 30 trillion cells, 78 organs, and 600 muscles that need daily attention. Though the brain is the number one organ because it controls the center of the nervous system, you need to distinguish between the ally's and enemies of your body. An article published in 2014 by Cornell University stated that when parasite worms invade muscle tissue white blood cells called eosinophil rush to the scene to stop the body from launching a chemical attack on the worm, enabling the parasite to make a home within the muscle. The earliest known parasite in a human was the lung fluke around 5900 BC. How it affects us in 2022 and beyond is the fact that they evolve, but they must be removed internally and externally. There are herbal remedies to remove some parasites, but to be rid of them all takes daily monitoring. Not treating them can possibly make you immobilized on many occasions.

I read articles of athletes suddenly not being able to get out of bed, who after certain testing find an infestation of parasites holding them back. There is a procedure that some scoff at yet works called plate zapping, parasite zapper, or zapper machine. By systematically destroying parasites, we eliminate the cause and not the symptoms of potential disease. Every live organism emits a unique and specific frequency that, if we were able to kind of jam signal of, wouldn't be able to function and would die. The devices talked about above use frequency or electric waves to remove pathogen organisms from our bodies. There are devices that use 9v DC power or on 32 KHz of frequency. All parasites have their own frequency and being that there could be six million species of parasites, a wide range at certain duration can kill them all for a day. Your whole body is made of live matter, so it shouldn't be a surprise to you. There are different types of devices, but the standard device has two copper handles for each hand where copper has been known to enable an electric current to pass over into your body, where it kills all the pathogen organisms. An alternative to copper handles is gel pad electrodes, where you just place the electrodes on your skin. Whichever device you use, the procedure is the same: You would do three seven-minute zapping intervals, each with a twenty- to thirty-minute rest period.

Here's the process:

First time, you do a seven-minute zapping session followed by a twenty-minute pause. In this first cycle or session, the device eliminates parasites by removing their outer membrane. This makes the parasite release all smaller parasites, bacteria and viruses that were living inside it.

Second time, do another seven-minute zapping session followed by a twenty-minute rest period or pause. During this session, we destroy harmful pathogens that were released during the first cycle.

The third and final session is the last cycle in which any other possible pathogens that were living inside the bacteria, viruses, and smaller parasites from the second cycle are removed. Now, you're done for the day. This whole procedure cleans your system for one day. Because we constantly eat the wrong foods on a daily basis, this is something you have to do every day or whenever possible.

But just like everything else, there are limitations here too. I recommend to not doing this treatment if you're pregnant or have a pacemaker because dealing with electrical frequencies may cause a bad reaction. You can't target pathogen organisms in hollow organs like the eyes, gut, or stomach with a zapper. For those areas, you need herbal remedies. You ideally should do this procedure every morning. Understand that conventional medicine may have its place, but it usually just focuses on the symptoms and not the cause. Gel electrodes allow for an easier use of the device, which is also compatible with copper bands should you switch them with copper handles, should you wish to switch them with electrodes. You may feel drowsy, which is a good thing, indicating things are getting out of your system and you just need recovery time. Never use it while driving. You also may feel thirsty and so stay hydrated. To avoid skin irritation, some may want wrist straps for your ankle as a second location. In terms of the electrodes, you can use the zapper just about anywhere on your body with the exception of your face for cosmetic reasons that may have a rare case where might provoke a seizure from using that area, only if someone is prone to seizures already. Don't use devices on open wounds, genitals, rectum, or front of the neck. The electrode style shouldn't matter for effectiveness. The metal tubes provide the best conductivity and the wristbands offer the most convenience. The adhesive electrodes can be placed with the greatest precision, anywhere on the body. From a quantum physics level, you cannot electrocute yourself because your frequency is tremendously high compared to a microscopic parasites frequency. For herbal remedies, I suggest a liquid form black walnut hull (one drop in a half cup of distilled water), wormwood capsules with water (one capsule a day), and clove capsules with water (three a day).

Your muscle is a tissue that contracts, shortens, or moves; the fact is that there are 600 different muscles in your body, the three main ones being the cardiac muscle, which contracts the heart; the smooth or visceral muscle, which transports food and waste material to their proper place; and the skeletal muscle, which do all the movements of the body every day.

Breaking down your workouts into even simpler routine, you'd notice that there are only two types: Anaerobic training, requiring no oxygen or rather more intense, but for shorter duration, like during body building. Then there's weight training and isometrics, which uses resistance without weights. And aerobic training uses a lot of oxygen, like long-distance running, jogging, biking, and swimming.

The brain doesn't focus on velocity or how quick you lift the weight; it just focuses on the task itself. Here's how you can know the difference between the two: A bodybuilder focuses on definition and size in certain parts of the body. A weightlifter only focuses on strength or the most he/she can lift with no interest in definition.

As far as growing food, I always questioned the growth of food and how there are more accommodating approaches like rotating crops, which is growing different types of crops in the same area across a sequence of growing seasons. This reduces one's reliance one set of nutrients, pests, and weed pressure. Alternating crops kill certain pests' survival. Another idea is rearing sterilized insects and then releasing them in areas of a particular pest that causes problems. Breeding beneficial insects and then releasing them to prey on pests also helps. Even using birds instead of pesticides is another option. You can even go back to fertilizing seeds with fish, something that was practiced by the early American Indians who were originally black. This method would be better instead of using animal manure. Hence the term "You are what you eat."

In My Opinion, Homemade is the Best:

Lemonade

One cup of fresh squeezed lemon juice
One cup of raw honey
1 ½ quart of water
¼ tsp. Vitamin C crystals
Bring honey and water to a boil, and then add lemon juice and Vitamin C crystals. Let it cool and then refrigerate.

Honey Water

One gallon water
3 cups honey raw
1 tsp. ginger

¼ tsp. Vitamin C crystals
Combine honey with water to boil and then add ginger and Vitamin C crystals. Let it cool and then refrigerate.

Maple Milk Shake

Take one glass of almond milk. You can use any kind of milk you choose. If cow's milk, make sure it's sterilized.
2 tbsp. maple syrup
¼ tsp. Vitamin C crystals Blend the above and drink.

A Natural Sandwich

Whole grain or wheat bread
Avocado deseeded and sliced
Cucumber sliced/skinned
Tomato sliced

Lettuce (patted dry after rinsing)
You put the lettuce on first and last of the sandwich to keep it from being soggy, after topping with mayo or butter.

I can never understand any diet you put in front of me because I feel depriving yourself of anything that you love doesn't work. It just takes being invited to that one family holiday dinner and your diet will literally die, pun the phrase. You should eat anything you want. But you can learn to do homemade instead of takeout of that same food you want. I don't believe god would point to you and say you're going to get cancer, diabetes, hypertension, or stroke. I think we create our own demise based on our choices. A disease is inherited if you eat the same foods, think the same way, live under the same roof, and have the same habits of your family. My education about health bought me back to the animals of the forest. Have you ever seen a lion with glasses? A bear with false teeth? A gorilla with a hearing aid? Or any animal, besides us, needing a dialysis machine? These animals eat well and stay fit because they never break certain rules that we break daily. There's a lifestyle called natural hygiene, which has been around since 1830 and was promoted by Dr. Herbert M. Shelton. On this topic, toxic substances, which are poisonous wastes or metabolic imbalances, are mentioned. These are some of many ways that create diseases in the body. Toxins are usually found in the thighs, buttocks, midsection or stomach, upper arms, and under the chin. These are the fatty tissues. Toxins can be also found in muscles. You become obese or overweight or lethargic and tired from too much acid or toxins. Toxins can be from having food still in your body, which has not been digested because of bad food combination. Also, if you drink a beverage during a meal, whether wine or water, it's best to drink fifteen minutes before a meal so that it doesn't interfere with the normal digestive juices during your normal digestive cycle.

These principles will never change. Do what you like. As long as you know the consequences of your actions.

You shouldn't combine these foods: Fish and rice, chicken and noodles, eggs and toast, cheese and bread, cereal and milk. These combinations create an enormous amount of acid, which cause arthritis in the long run in the joints. Just a year of combining these foods can do damage. Those foods can sit in your system for days, weeks, and even months. It's possible due to improper food combining. To make it easy for you, remember not to combine a protein (eggs, dairy, and nuts) with a starch (bread, rice, and pasta). A starch and a starch are good because they won't spoil each other in your stomach. But a protein and a protein are not good because they're too complex. Rice and beans has been a good friend during hard times. Though heavy, it agrees with my stomach. Tortilla and beans is digestible, along with an avocado sandwich with corn chips. Further examples of a toxic body is gray hair (I always considered it a deficiency), nervous outburst (I personally don't blame bipolar for this one), dark circles under the eyes, premature lines, ulcers, and stress, which, I feel, have nothing to do with aging. A lot of things people associate to aging are stereotypes, and people that grow "old" just learned to accept their demise. Three areas you must take care of at all times are your brain, kidneys, and liver because the most well-known diseases have been found in these three areas.

You don't get protein from taking protein. Let me say that again: you don't get protein from taking protein. It has to be broken down in your body a certain way. Your body makes protein inside your system from amino acids, which are found in certain foods. Animal protein is not human protein that your body needs. There are twenty-three kinds of amino acids. Fifteen of them the body makes and the remaining eight you get from outside sources—from fruits, vegetables, nuts, seeds, and sprouts. The fuel from your body is made from carbohydrates which is an organic compound. Fats supply energy and change into fuel when there's no carbohydrates left in the body. Don't forget to add super foods to your lifestyle, which are organic greens. Seek out places where their meat and poultry are naturally and organically grazed with no chemicals. Eat a small portion of meat daily if at all. Meat, duck, and pork are the hardest things to digest. The best way to get calcium, still in 2022 and beyond, is by taking in organically grown green leafy vegetables, raw nuts, and sesame seeds. Anything cooked loses its nutritional value.

To explain the acid in your body: Your body has a pH (public health) balance. It's a degree of acid or alkaline. The pH levels are between zero (total acid) to fourteen (total alkaline). Cancer cannot survive in an alkaline state. A level of seven is neutral. This is measured in your blood. A reading of 7.35 to 7.40 pH means your blood is slightly alkaline. At 7.0, it means there could be a problem if not monitored because the more acid in the body, the more the body will keep water in to neutralize the body, which causes weight gain.

As a side note: agave nectar, stevia (a plant), raw honey, brown sugar and licorice root liquid are good natural sweeteners.

Niacin (flush, which you'll feel tingly), niacinamide (non-flush), Ginko biloba, and cognition have been known to open blood vessels to allow oxygen to the brain for better memory.

Six Types of Hormones That Rule Your Body:

Melatonin: This controls your sleep/wake cycle. Also, in theory, it affects your biological clock or pineal gland, a small, pea shaped gland in the brain.

Progesterone (female hormones) and testosterone (male hormones)

Cortisol (the stress hormone)

Insulin: Those with Type1 and Type 2 diabetes have high blood sugar. The hormone insulin is necessary for the cells in your body to properly use the glucose in your bloodstream.

Estrogen: Estrogen is critical to bone health and having less of it is associated with osteoporosis, a condition where your bones become more fragile or porous. As menopause approaches, women's bodies produce less estrogen.

A side note:

As you build the inside and work on the outside, there is a law of physics: You can train hard (intensity), you can train long (duration), but you can't do both because you'd be dead from exhausted resources.

The number one cause of death is famine, which is lack of food. Second cause of death is malnutrition, which is due to a weak immune system, which is also lack of food. That is why after you eat something, you may still feel hungry.

What Does This Have to Do With health?
Everything!
Before you can ever be good on the outside
You must first start from within

The Mental Stage

"Now faith is being sure of what we hope for and certain of what we do not see. This is what the ancients were commended for. By faith, we understand that the universe was formed at God's command, so that what is seen was not made out of what was visible."

Hebrews 11: 1–3

The power of visualization has help through the years. It is a scientific fact that your brain cannot tell the difference on what's real and what's not. Only one's perception of a situation is what matters. To be your own greatest hero, just look in the mirror and say, "I am my greatest hero." It's really that simple. Just like the best things in life are free, the simplest thing can empower you. The conscious mind can only do one to two tasks at a time; the subconscious can absorb an endless amount of information at once. Unfortunately, we experience more bad than good and everything we experience stays in the file of your brain. If you feel any pain, physical or mental, do not talk about them. Do not! Do not think about them. Do Not! It is the repetition of going over and over it that keeps it there. It is repetition to not talk about them. It is repetition to not think about them that makes them go away.

Ivan Pavloff studied the principles of proper food combining. He was famous for showing the effects of anchors and how sounds can change a person's state or feeling. Psychology is the scientific study of the mind and behavior. He practiced this on dogs using a bell and a piece of meat where he would ring a bell as the dogs were salivating while looking at the meat. He would just ring the bell for minutes at a time. After the dogs ate the meat, he would just ring a bell, and the dogs would start to salivate even after they'd finished eating, by just hearing the bell's sound alone. This is how the mind can be conditioned.

Before WWII in Paris, France, there was a place that taught autosuggestion using phonograph records, which were played over and over again, and listeners heard any subject they wanted. Whichever record was picked, it gave them the repeated suggestions, if they were in good health, let's say, regardless of their age, race, and gender—that they had the power to overcome their difficulties and that they would receive help in other ways, even if they appeared to be physically and mentally alone. For hundreds of years, mothers were taught to talk to their babies, from the time a woman was pregnant, by listening to baroque classical music, to the time their children were born and while their children were asleep; the mothers would repeat things like their kids were going to develop good habits and be good people. Due to the fact that the children were asleep, the suggestions were directed to their subconscious mind.

People may oppose me on this, but when you command your neurotransmitters in your head to create an image in your brain, that's a physically direct command. Because you're telling your mind what to do. When you let the world or society dictate what you can and cannot do, that's an indirect mental command because you're not exerting it yourself but you're accepting what's being said. In other words, you're simply buying what they're selling.

With social media everybody wants to know everything about everybody, because most are scared of the unknown. Life would be pretty boring if you knew everything that was going to happen to you before it happens to you. We all need that sense of mystery. Besides, knowing everything about everybody goes against The Six Human Needs: You really need all of them to be "Happy": certainty, uncertainty or variety, unique, acceptance or unity, growth, and love (of yourself and the world).

This subject has been talked about for eons. With age, it can be a blessing or burden, based on your reality and your models of the world. If we ever meet and discuss the subject of age, I would simply say, "Age is nothing; belief is everything. Youth is energy and focus. That's all it is. It's not about age, but about energy and spirit. When the spirit is willing, the flesh is strong. Not weak, but strong. But you must work at it. A strong spirit can move mountains. When you give something a name, you give it limitation. Choose to be limitless. Be treated as a person. Not a liability. With age, you either do or do not, there is no try." If you put 100 30-year-olds in a room, you're going to get a hundred different interpretations of what 30 means to them. It's the same if you put in the room a 100 40-, 50-, 60- year-olds, and so on. No matter what chronological age you are, you're still a man or woman who's a child of God. Facts: Forget the numbers for a moment as far as your age, weight, location, income, etc. is concerned, and just look at yourself by getting to the root of it. You're made of pure energy that never dies but just changes form.

As far as the theories out there, the two common ones are Damaged Theories and Program Theories. According to Damaged Theories, damage occurs inside cells over time, caused by things called free radicals. These are atoms or molecules with impaired electrons in their outer shell that steal from other molecules to restore their balance. As a result, they spread and multiply, destroying healthy cells in the process. Oxygen is the most widely spread free radical in the body. Which is why we must breathe in and out because it turns to carbon dioxide, a poisonous gas. Without antioxidants to keep it in check free radicals would form disease or chronic illnesses.

In Programmed Theories, the idea is that aging happens because of a genetic clock that decides when cells no longer operate or produce. To create an alkaline state in your body, you can drink a liter of filtered or osmosis reversed water with lemon daily but don't eat genetically modified (GMO) organisms; that's not natural. So going GMO-free or with no GMO would be organically made corn, beets, zucchini, summer squash, radishes, and Hawaiian papaya.

There was a study at Columbia University where people in their seventies and eighties were involved in weight training. The demand that the participants were doing were so great that it was putting pressure on their pituitary gland thus creating a growth hormone making them biologically younger and stronger.

Organic wheat grass and alfalfa leaves help rid the body of acids when taken daily.

We're in the twenty-first century and still the top ten causes of death are heart disease, cancer, cerebrovascular disease (stroke), chronic lung disease, accidents, pneumonia/influenza, diabetes mellitus, HIV infection, suicide (which was rising during the pandemic), and liver diseases.

Putting together this book taught me a lot of things:

If you think what you need is not there, find it. If you can't find it, make it. If you cannot make it, find someone who can. If can't find someone, get credit. If you can't get credit, go out and do something that someone will pay you for, so you can pay for what you need. There are no but's too big that they cannot be moved.

What Does This Have To Do with Health?
Everything!
We are thoughts that became things
So use everything you got just to be…

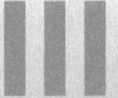

The Emotional Stage

"Finally, Brothers and Sisters, whatever is true, whatever is noble, whatever is right, whatever is pure, whatever is lovely, whatever is admirable— if anything is excellent or praiseworthy—think about such things. Whatever you have learned or received or heard from me, or seen in me-put it into practice. And the God of peace will be with you."

Philippians 4:4

Emotion is created by motion. Many times through trial and error, I didn't like working out but I liked the results, which kept me going to create a habit. You may relate to that. When it comes to training, you may have to play tricks with your brain to motivate yourself to work out. I knew people in business and in entertainment industry that needed an "edge" and would use performance enhancing drugs or some kind of short cut for instant gratification. I came close to doing that, but it went against my principles. Plus, when I learned my history I learned from the mistakes of others and the biggest mistake that was missing was discipline and a code of conduct. I decided to adopt those. You need passion to start and succeed in your healthier routine. To help those to be motivated even more. All the time while working in a hospital, people would always tell me one of the two things: "Don't grow old," and "I wish I could do my life over." Throughout the pandemic regret was the dominate force. Decide to be healthier for whatever time you have in this world. It's funny that people I read about and succeeded said they lived each day as though it was their last. As a result, they lived and achieved for much longer than they anticipated.

I have a gift of perception where I could literally see where I was going if I didn't try something. That's the true measure of a man. It's not whether you win or lose but that you try. I thought of what would happen if I didn't stay healthy. Thoughts, words, and images would come to me as if God was showing me the way. So to every generation I'd tell this: A want can be compromised, a need cannot. You must need to be "healthy," whatever that means to you. Look at the ones around you, be honest with yourself, and ask if you want to settle with what life gave you.

"Goals weigh ounces, but regret weighs tons." You must be almost "obsessed," like breathing. To deal with challenges that will affect your mood along the way, there are different techniques I discovered to live for another day:

Laughter is the best medicine. Not fake ones to wallow in misery, but those that are a result of watching funny movies or books; those can bring your body into an alkaline state. A grin is a second way to change from a horrible state. I do what I call wingspans: Choose a place you have enough space to first put your hand in a prayer position and then pull them apart as far as possible, creating this huge wingspan, while stretching your fingers out as well. Now, bringing your hands back in to a prayer position and repeating this: out, in, out, and in about ten times. The purpose of doing this is to change your state. Everything we do is a means (person, place, or thing) to an end (a result), so realize it is what you make it. You can be a ship tossed around with no sail or steering wheel and just float your life away, or you can be a nuclear-powered vessel that can go anywhere it wants to. The choice is yours: the placebo or the cure!

What Does That Have To Do with Health?
Everything!
Without emotional conviction,
Life will overcome you until you overcome life

IV

//

The Spiritual Stage

"I Thought, 'Age should speak; advanced years should teach wisdom.' But it is the spirit in man, the breath of the Almighty that gives him understanding."

Job 32: 7&8

The ancient ones knew the connection between you and the divine. They knew that buried deep in your perceptions and self-imposed limitations is a spirit of unlimited possibility. You create with your own reality the conditions you will face. You limit with your fear your true desires. You destroy with your own blame the direction of your destiny. The ancient ones knew that with your mind and emotions, you would master your fate. If you believe the blood of the ancient ones runs through your veins then you have the same knowledge. Each day, millions of creative talented people sit wasting away, perhaps losing their job or home, not having any money but still having the power to think of an apparatus or creative idea for that to become a seed that turns into a tree. That turns into a forest. That makes the buildings and homes from the wood. Have depth of vision and create your own luck. As this book revealed, there are four stages in life you go through: the physical stage, mental stage, emotional stage, and spiritual stage. When separate they are good, but together they're invincible. In a world of chaos, there must be order. In a world of hysteria, there must be serenity. Invest in meditation for inner peace. One of the true realities of life is five, ten, or twenty years from now you will arrive. The question is where? Create a "where" that's self-imposed and something to live for. The best way to deal with a problem is before it ever comes up. So be proactive or prepared daily instead of reactive to things you may not be able to control. Because you still have the power to choose your own attitude.

Something had happened because of which I wasn't going to write this book. I decided to not just finish it, but add to it as inspiration. It was March 22, 2022. For some reason, something told me to get up at midnight, the start of the day. No matter what time I would wake up, I would do my regular routine. I would first drink a liter of filtered water, followed by options of either taking chlorophyll (a green plant liquidated), organic wheat grass or whole food supplements in a concentrated form. Then, I would work on my book. An hour later, I would drink juice to rejuvenate and cleanse my system. No rule on how I juice. Variety is the spice of life. An hour after that, I ate breakfast and continued writing my book. I showered and dressed up thinking I'd go running. It was around 6 a.m. when all of a sudden I heard a thump downstairs. I lived in a two-family private house that my stepdad owned. I rented upstairs while he lived downstairs. I went downstairs to see if things were alright. I knocked on the door but got no answer. Luckily, there was a window through his door. I looked in and saw my stepdad's legs outside the front of his room. I yelled, "He's on the floor. He's on the floor." Right away his son came out of his own room in the house. He went to check on Stepdad. "Call 911," he said to me. I couldn't get in his door yet so I went was inspirational and revelations were deep. But there was a phrase that kept my sanity and helped me live for another day:

"Now faith is being sure of what we hope for and certain of what we do not see. This is what the ancients were commended for. By faith we understand that the universe was formed at God's command. So that is seen is not made out of what is visible."

Hebrews 11:1–3

What that means to me is that everything begins with a thought. That we are thoughts that became things. So I decided to use all my thoughts to become a great thing. So through trial and error, I felt like Thomas Edison, who successfully found 10,000 ways that it would not work until he found one way that it did, which is how I got here. I rose from the ashes of my past to become a fiery Phoenix. And I end this speech with a poem that a great man told me years ago. A poem by Elsa Beech Wheeler:

> "With every rising of the sun
> Think of your life as just begun
> The past is cancelled. Buried deep
> All yesterdays there. Let them sleep
> Concern yourself with but today
> Grasp it and teach to obey
> You were well and plan since time began
> Today has been a friend of man
> You and today and a soul sublime
> And a great heritage of time
> With God and self to bind the twain
> Go forth, brave soul. Obtain, obtain"

For years, I've been rehearsing this speech with no real money and no real friends. But just a dream and asked God if I would ever tell my story to anyone, and today God gave me the answer.

Thank You.

People I Admire

Lee Haney: An all American Bodybuilder standing 5 feet 11 inches tall. He shares the all-time record for Mr. Olympia titles, having eight at the time, tied with Ronnie Coleman. I admired him for his consistency and determination.

Michael Anthony Jerome "Spud" Webb: An all-American former professional basketball NBA player, standing 5 feet 6 inches tall. He blew me away when he won the 1986 Slam Dunk Contest, being a "Little Giant." I admired him for making "the impossible" quite possible.

Billy Wayne Blanks: An American fitness personality and martial artist, standing 6 feet tall. I admired him for his marketability in business and in life.

Michael "Jeffrey" Jordan: A former American NBA professional player, from Brooklyn, NY, standing 6 feet 6 inches tall. I admired his "To Not Accept Not Trying," a philosophy and a good book, as well as his other book, "Air."

William D. Dickerson: A cousin whose life was cut short, never letting him make it professionally in basketball who could have potentially been one of the greatest players of all time. He personally taught me to be disciplined and that to be the best you have to train like the best. He also taught me that health is 90% mental and 10% physical.

Julius Winfield "Erving" II: An American former ABA and NBA

professional player, standing at 6 feet and 7 inches tall, from East Meadows, NY. I knew about him at the pinnacle of his career while he played for the Philadelphia 76ers. I admired him for his workout ethic being discipline.

Kyrie "Andrew" Irving: An American NBA professional player, standing at 6 feet 2 inches tall. I admire him for standing for what he believes in.

Bruce "Jun-Fan" Lee: An American martial artist, from Hong Kong, China, standing at 5 feet 8 inches tall. I admire him for not only revolutionizing martial arts but also beating the odds against opposition in the entertainment world.

Colin "Rand" Kaepernick: An American civil rights activist and former football quarterback, who played six seasons with the San Francisco 49ers in the NFL. Standing 6 feet 4 inches tall. I admire him for his determination, sincerity, and just being "real."

Organic Farming:

This is big business and well-practiced around the globe. The strongest organic farming is still known to be in North America and in the Western Hemisphere. Organic farming is also big in Europe, but the greatest dedicated area has been known to be Australia. A number of big producers have also been in India and the Falkland Islands. After WW II, everything was being internationalized and just expanding.

Health Related Organizations

American Cancer Society: Established in 1913 in Atlanta, GA. It's nationwide dedicated to eliminating cancer.

The Centers for Disease Control and Prevention (CDC): A health agency of the United States. Founded in 1946 in Atlanta, GA, it's a federal agency.

The World Health Organization (WHO): A specialized agency of The United Nations, which is responsible for the international public health and was established in 1948 in Geneva, Switzerland.

The U.S. Food and Drug Administration: A federal agency that's a part of The Department of Health and Human Services and was founded in 1906 in Silver Springs, MD. It is responsible for protecting the public by ensuring the safety, efficiency, and security of human and veterinary drugs and biological products.

American Public Health Association (APHA): The oldest and most diverse public health professionals in the world, which was established in 1872 in Washington, DC.

The Carter Center: This organization conducts health programs around the world to help fill many of the vacuums in global health. A non-governmental organization founded in 1982 by former president, Jimmy Carter, it helps resolve conflicts.

CVS Health (Consumer Value Stores): They're combined with Aetna, a health insurance company. Founded in 1963, CVS is a leading health solutions company headquartered in Lowell, Massachusetts.

National Academy of Sciences (NAS): A private non-profit organization that was founded in 1863 in Washington, D.C.

The Academy of Nutrition and Diabetics (Formerly the American Dietetic Association): It's the world's largest organization of food and nutrition professionals which was established in 1917 in Chicago, IL.

The Difference between Alzheimer's and Dementia:

Alzheimer's disease, also called senile dementia, destroys memory and other important mental functions. It eventually wipes out everything. However, dementia by itself is not a specific disease but interferes with daily cognitive functioning.

With this, selective things may be erased.

References

Before The Mayflower, Lerone Bennet Jr.

Man's Search for Meaning, Viktor Frankl

The Game of Life and How to Play It, Florence Schovel Shinn

Blacks in Science, Jan Van Sertima

The Cure for All Diseases, Hulda Regehr Clark

Ultimate Anti-Aging Program, Gary Null

I Can't Accept Not Trying, Michael Jordan

Acts of Faith, Iyanla Vanzant

The Magic of Believing, Claud M. Bristol

Diet for a New America, John Robbins

Back To Eden, Jethro Kloss

Sports Nutrition Guidebook, Nancy Clark

Powernomics, Dr. Claud Anderson

Fit for Life, Harvey and Marilyn Diamond

IP6 Natures Revolutionary Cancer-Fighter, Abulkalam M. Shamsuddin

Static Contraction Training, Peter Sisco & John Little

About the Author

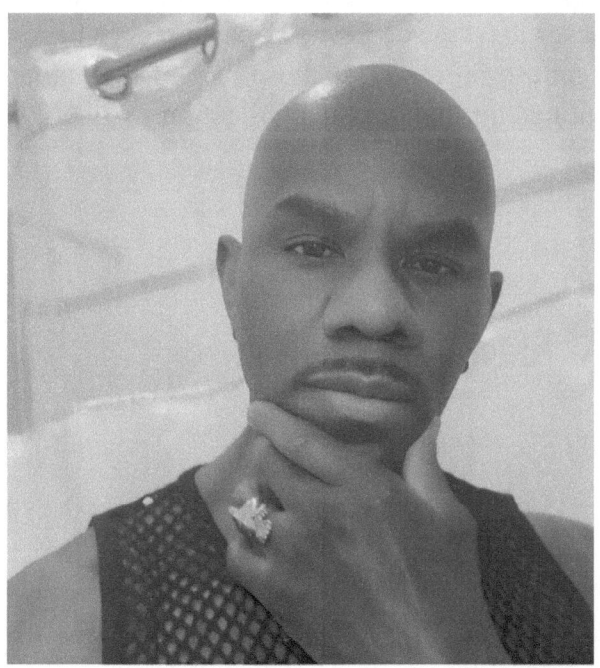

Pbody Blaque aka Dwayne M., is a Black Foundational American author, entrepreneur, poet, and fitness enthusiast. He learned about health at the lowest point of people's lives. With the chance at learning conventional medicine, by seeing many of his love ones die at the hands of institutions, he decided to switch to holistic natural medicine. He believes that regardless of the ailment, the whole body, and not just the symptoms, must be tended to. His dear Aunt Elizabeth's death devastated him to the point where it changed his view of life. He said, "I don't care how rich, popular, or 'powerful' you are. If you don't have health, good health, you have nothing." He currently resides in New York.

"I guarantee you will think outside the box after reading this book."

— Pbody Blaque

Pbody Blaque is transparent with the reader in this self-help guide. With the goal of connecting to all those committed to enhancing their reality, Pbody showcases that "the dedication" portion goes beyond just names. Seekers will get a brief on all of those part of the author's journey as they are mentioned throughout the publication.

www.ingramcontent.com/pod-product-compliance
Lightning Source LLC
Chambersburg PA
CBHW020339130626
46549CB00003B/1213